High Blood Pressure:

40 Super-food that will naturally lower your blood pressure

High Blood Pressure

Author

Arnold Yates

Table of Contents

Introduction 3

Chapter One: 5

What Causes High Blood Pressure 5

Chapter Two: 16

How to Prevent High Blood Pressure 16

Chapter 3 21

Low Sodium Cooking Tips 21

Chapter 4 27

Meal planning 27

Chapter 5 30

Breakfast 30

Chapter 6 33

Lunch and Dinner 33

Chapter 7 37

Dessert 37

Chapter 8 39

High Blood Pressure

40 Super Foods That Will Naturally Lower Your Blood Pressure 39

Chapter 9 54

Bonus Juicing Recipes 54

Chapter 10 56

Relaxing Techniques 56

Conclusion 62

Introduction

Blood pressure refers to the force exerted on the arterial walls when the heart pumps blood. The large amount of force on the walls of the arteries over a sustained period of time is referred to as high blood pressure.

High blood pressure or hypertension is one of the most common health problems associated with lifestyle choices. The problem is more common in older adults than in the younger generations.

Recent estimates by the American Heart Association (AHA) indicate that 65 million American adults which translate to about 1 in 3 people have high blood pressure. The condition is more common and more serious in African American populations compared to the Caucasian population.

High Blood Pressure

High blood pressure is equally prevalent in other parts of the world and it is estimated that it kills one billion people worldwide. With the modern lifestyle punctuated by poor eating and sedentary lifestyles, the prevalence of high blood pressure is gradually rising.

Normal blood pressure is denoted as 120/80 mmHg. The higher number (120) refers to systolic blood pressure when the heart forcefully pumps blood through the arteries. The lower figure gives a reading of the diastolic pressure which is the pressure when the heart rests between beats.

If the blood pressure reading is consistently slightly higher than 120/80 mmHg, the condition is referred to as prehypertension which places people at high risk of getting high blood pressure. Steps have to be taken to prevent high blood pressure from developing into the fully blown condition.

High blood pressure is diagnosed from a reading higher than 140/90 mmHg and is often referred to as the silent killer, and with good reason. It will most often go undetected and it doesn't have openly identifiable symptoms. Medical professionals classify high blood pressure in two stages: Stage I high blood pressure from readings of 140-159/90-99 and Stage II high blood pressure from readings 160/100 or higher. High blood pressure is linked to other serious health conditions such as stroke, coronary heart disease, kidney failure, heart attack, and other health problems and risks.

High Blood Pressure

It is important for people with high blood pressure to understand the condition and the ways through which they can effectively manage the condition and also prevent the condition where appropriate. The information is also useful for caregivers and people who live with the high blood pressure patients.

Chapter One:

What Causes High Blood Pressure

The exact causes of high blood pressure are not well known but a number of factors have been identified in the development of the condition.

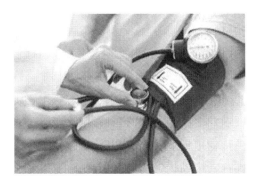

Fig: Taking blood pressure readings

There are two types of high blood pressure depending on the cause.

High Blood Pressure

I. Primary/Essential hypertension – the high blood pressure that does not have an identifiable cause. It can however be linked to a number of risk factors and will develop gradually over the years.

II. Secondary hypertension – it is the high blood pressure caused by an underlying health. Secondary hypertension will often appear suddenly and is linked to higher blood pressure readings compared to essential hypertension. The most common conditions associated with secondary high blood pressure are congenital defects of blood vessels, obstructive sleep apnea, thyroid problems, kidney problems and adrenal gland problems.

We have a look at the common causes of high blood pressure.

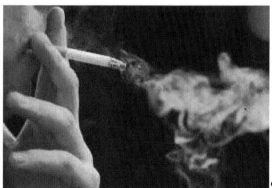

a) Smoking – the use of tobacco either by smoking or chewing is known to cause a temporal rise in blood pressure levels. Nicotine alongside other chemicals in tobacco will over the long term destroy arterial walls

High Blood Pressure

making the arteries to narrow. The resultant effect is that blood pressure tends to rise. Similar effects are also caused by secondhand smoke.

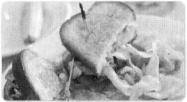

A diet high in sodium and low in nutritional value puts you at higher risk for HBP.

b) Diet – majority of the fast food restaurants as well as baked food carry a dual threat of causing obesity due to high calorie content and the threat of carrying too much salt since most ingredients are processed foods. These two threats have a profound effect on blood pressure levels.

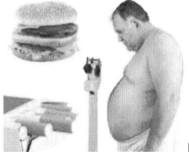

c) Being overweight or obese increases the risk of developing high blood pressure. A body mass index (BMI) between 25 and 30 is considered overweight. A body mass index over 30 is considered obese. About two-thirds of U.S. adults are overweight or obese. About one in three U.S. children ages 2 to 19 are overweight or obese. Excess weight increases the strain on the heart, raises blood cholesterol and triglyceride

High Blood Pressure

levels, and lowers HDL (good) cholesterol levels. It can also make diabetes more likely to develop. Losing as little as 10 to 20 pounds can help lower your blood pressure and your heart disease risk. To successfully and healthfully lose weight—and keep it off—most people need to subtract about 500 calories per day from their diet to lose about 1 pound per week.

d) Lack of physical activity increases the risk of obesity and high blood pressure. People who are not physically active tend to have higher heart rates. Today, daily routines are characterized by hours of sitting at a desk using computers and browsing the internet, watching television shows, and using countless labor-saving devices which in effect means that you can easily fall into inactivity. But taking charge of your fitness by engaging in exercise may be one of the best ways of preventing high blood pressure.

e) 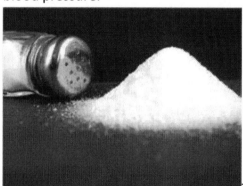 Too much salt is associated with the high incidence of essential hypertension. Salt makes your body hold on to

High Blood Pressure

water. The extra water stored in your body raises your blood pressure. Hypertensive people are sensitive to high amounts of salt that raises blood pressure due to fluid retention.

f) 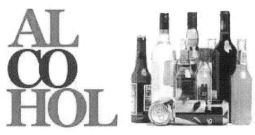 Too much alcohol consumption damages the heart. It should not be more than two drinks a day for men and more than one drink a day for women. Repeated binge drinking can lead to long-term increases in blood pressure. Alcohol also contains lots of calories and may contribute to unwanted weight gain, a risk factor for high blood pressure.

g) High stress levels lead to temporary increase in blood pressure and may exacerbate problems in people who already have high blood pressure. In stressful situations, the body produces hormones that temporarily increase your blood pressure by causing your heart to beat faster and your blood vessels to narrow.

h) Gender is another cause of high blood pressure. More adult men compared to women have high blood pressure. However, younger women between the ages of 18 and 59 years are more likely compared to men of similar age to be aware of and

High Blood Pressure

seek treatment for blood pressure. Women older than 60 years have the same likelihood as men of being aware of and seeking treatment for high blood pressure. The only difference is that the control of blood pressure is lower in women over 60 years than it is in men of the same age group.

i) Genetic factors –Genetic factors likely play some role in high blood pressure, heart disease, and other related conditions. Numerous genes have been identified that cause high blood pressure especially those that alter the renin-angiotensin system. However, it is also likely that people with a family history of high blood pressure share common environments and other potential factors that increase their risk.

The risk for high blood pressure can increase even more when heredity combines with unhealthy lifestyle choices, such as smoking cigarettes and eating an unhealthy diet.

j) Family history of high blood pressure – you are most likely to get high blood pressure if other members of your family have, or have had, high blood pressure.

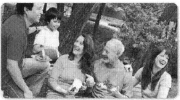

Eye color isn't your only inherited trait. You may also share a risk for HBP.

Family members have a lot in common. They share genes, behaviors, lifestyles, and environments that can influence their health and their risk for high

High Blood Pressure

blood pressure . High blood pressure can run in a family, and your risk for high blood pressure can increase based on your age and your race or ethnicity.

k) Menopause – Blood pressure generally increases after menopause. The onset of menopause is associated with hormonal changes that tend to cause or are associated with high blood pressure. Menopause-related hormonal changes in women can lead to weight gain and make your blood pressure more reactive to salt in your diet. Additionally, some of the common types of hormone therapy used for menopause may contribute to increases in blood pressure levels.

l) Lack of or too little vitamin D in your diet can affect an enzyme produced by your kidneys that regulate blood pressure leading to high blood pressure. Potassium affects the balance of fluids in the body.

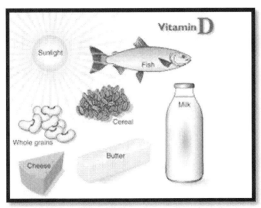

Fig: Source of Vitamin D

High Blood Pressure

Insufficient potassium intake in diet can lead to the accumulation of too much sodium in the cells leading to retention of fluid and causing high blood pressure. Too much potassium can be harmful especially in people with kidney disorders. Chronic kidney disease leads to elevated blood pressure. People with kidney disease are much more likely to develop high blood pressure, heart disease, or have a stroke.

m) Adrenal and thyroid disorders are recognized as causes of secondary high blood pressure. People with hypothyroidism have twice the greater risk of developing hypertension compared to normal people. Low amounts of thyroid hormone can slow heartbeat which affects pumping strength and blood vessel wall flexibility. Both will lead to a rise in blood pressure levels.

n) Sleep apnea is a sleep condition associated with high blood pressure. Sleep apnoea is characterized by cessation of breathing due to block airways.

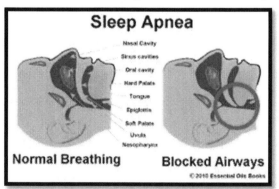

High Blood Pressure

Fig: Sleep apnoea, a sleep condition causes high blood pressure

These apnea episodes produce rise in systolic and diastolic pressure that keep mean blood pressure levels elevated at night. Hypertension may also be caused by sympathetic nervous system over-activity and alterations in vascular function and structure caused by oxidant stress and inflammation.

o) Race – high blood pressure is more common among the black population often developing at an earlier age than it does in whites. Serious complications, such as stroke, heart attack and kidney failure are also more common in blacks. Other people at greater risk of high blood pressure are people from South Asia.

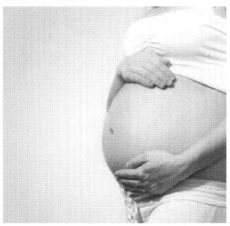

Fig: Pregnancy is linked to high blood presssure

p) Pregnant women are at high risk of high blood pressure cause by factors such as physical inactivity, poor lifestyle choices e.g. smoking, maternal age, carrying more than one baby, being overweight, first

High Blood Pressure

time pregnancies, and a previous history of high blood pressure.

q) Women who take birth control pills are at high risk of high blood pressure. Birth control pills and the hormonal birth control devices contain hormones that may increase your blood pressure in different ways such as narrowing smaller blood vessels. The majority of all these birth control pills, patches, and vaginal rings come with the warning that high blood pressure may be a side effect.

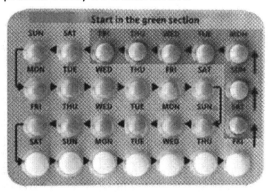

Fig: Birth control pills

It is important that women speak to their health practitioners when deciding to take hormonal contraceptives and to get regular checkups to screen for serious health problems.

r) Older age - the risk of high blood pressure increases as people grow older. As older adults live longer, they may suffer from one or many chronic diseases. They may also have a health problem that can lead

High Blood Pressure

to another condition or injury if not properly managed.

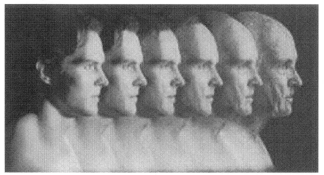

From about 45 years of age, high blood pressure is more common in men whereas the risk of high blood pressure in women tends to increase after the age of 65 years. The highest risk of high blood pressure is in the older people who suffer from obesity, diabetes, and chronic kidney disease

s) Medications – there are a number of medications that cause an increase in blood pressure levels. Some of these drugs are recreational drugs such as cocaine and amphetamines, the combined oral contraceptive pill, steroid medication, some over-the-counter cough and cold remedies, non-steroidal anti-inflammatory drugs (NSAIDs) such as ibuprofen and naproxen, herbal remedies that contain liquorice, and selective serotonin-noradrenaline reuptake inhibitor (SSNRI) antidepressants e.g. venlafaxine.

These medications may change the way your body controls fluid and salt balances, others may cause blood vessels to constrict, or yet others may impact the working of the renin-angiotensin-aldosterone system leading to high blood pressure.

These drugs should be avoided or used under the direction of your doctor following a review of your health status.

Chapter Two:

How to Prevent High Blood Pressure

The prevention of high blood pressure commences with a number of activities or interventions that surround lifestyle choices and maintaining healthy body weight.

The combination of the following steps will put you on the path to good health that is free of high blood pressure.

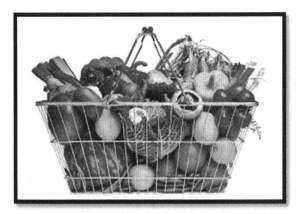

Fig: Healthy diet choices

High Blood Pressure

Follow a healthy eating plan that is characterized by a diet of green vegetables, fresh fruits, whole grains, legumes, fish rich in omega-3 fats, and low fat dairy products. Foods to be avoided include red meat, sugary foods and beverages and coconut oil.

- Limit the intake of salt (sodium) at low but healthy level to keep the body in a healthy state. It means that you choose and prepare foods that are lower in salt content or without added salt. You can also limit the use of the salt shaker at the dinner table.

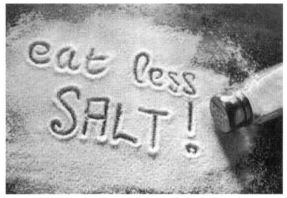

Fig: Eating lesser amounts of salt will prevent high blood pressure

Overall, the consumption of sodium should not exceed 2300 mg per day.

The dietary approaches to stop hypertension (DASH) plans are designed for high blood pressure patients. The DASH eating plan emphasizes that people consume whole grains, fruits and vegetables all of which are low in cholesterol, fat, and salt. It also emphasizes the importance of an active lifestyle.

High Blood Pressure

- Managing stress though relaxing and creating the ability to cope with problems will guarantee both physical and emotional health.

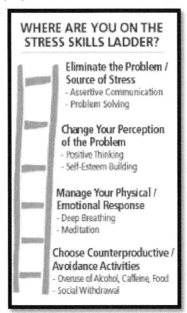

Fig: Ways of dealing with stress

Methods of reducing stress can include physical activity, relaxing, listening to music, practicing yoga and meditation.

- Being and remaining physically active reduces the risk of high blood pressure and other health problems.

High Blood Pressure

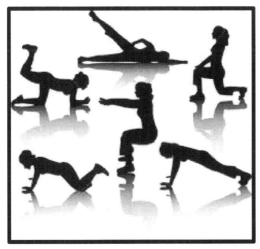

Fig: Physical activity helps maintain heart health

Consult your doctor on whether it is safe for you to engage in different kinds of physical activities. The threshold is for people to participate in moderate-intensity aerobic exercises for at least 2 hours and 30 minutes each week, or vigorous-intensity aerobic exercises for at least 1 hour and 15 minutes per week.

- Maintaining healthy body weight is important for the control of high blood pressure and for the reduction of the risk of heart disease.

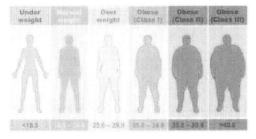

Fig: Maintaining a healthy BMI will keep high blood pressure at bay

High Blood Pressure

People who are overweight or obese should try to lose weight to improve on important factors such as blood pressure readings, to lower LDL cholesterol and to increase HDL cholesterol.

The best indicator of being overweight or obese is the body mass index (BMI) which measures weight in relation to height. The healthy range is a BMI of between 18.5 and 24.9 and anything greater than 25 is either overweight or obese.

- Alcohol intake should be limited to the recommended levels per day. Excessive consumption of alcohol increases triglyceride levels, a type of fat found in blood, and will also raise blood pressure levels.

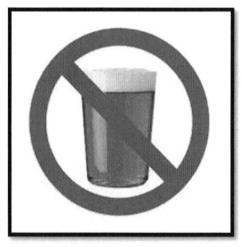

Fig: Regulate the intake of alcohol

Alcohol also contains excessive amounts of calories which lead to weight gain and predisposes people to high blood pressure.

High Blood Pressure

The threshold is men should not have more than two drinks containing alcohol a day whereas women should not have more than one drink containing alcohol a day. A drink represents 12 ounces of beer or 5 ounces of wine.

Chapter 3

Low Sodium Cooking Tips

With the American Diabetes Association indicating that the average person is consuming an equivalent of 3,400 mg of sodium per day against a recommended 2300 mg per day, it is important that people cut back on the consumption of sodium.

Low sodium consumption can be achieved by decreasing the amount of sodium in the diet. Low sodium diets are particularly important for people with high blood pressure and other heart diseases. By decreasing the amount of sodium in their diet, the hypertensive patients will be effectively reducing their risk of stroke or heart attacks.

The biggest source of sodium in diet is the processed foods as well as foods prepared in restaurants and other eateries. A big chunk of foods contain many hidden sources of calcium which makes it difficult for people to make healthy

High Blood Pressure

choices. The following tips will prove useful in the attempt to cut back on the amount of sodium in food.

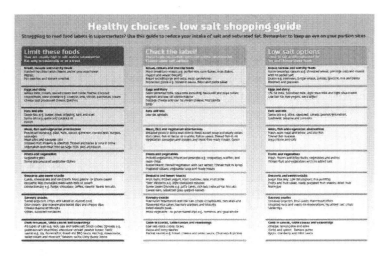

Fig: Low salt guide to cooking ingredients

Use fresh food instead of the processed foods. You should include fresh food such as dried beans, unsalted nuts and seeds, vegetables and fruits in your diet to replace the use of processed foods.

Other foods that can be included in their diet are whole grains such as brown rice, oats, wild rice, bulgur, quinoa, and whole grain barley that have not been prepared with salt.

These attempts will certainly help to reduce sodium intake and to increase the overall nutrient quality of prepared meals. The restaurant meals and processed food should be gradually eliminated from diet.

High Blood Pressure

Cook more at home to ensure that you are preparing a healthy meal. Eating out is the biggest cause of sodium loading with as little as the standard take away pack of a cheeseburger, a small serving of fries, and diet soda loading up to 950 mg of sodium.

By cooking at home, you have more control on what you will be preparing as a meal and eating. It begins with keeping the pantry, the refrigerator, and the freezer is stocked with lower-sodium options that will aid to prepare meals and to even prepare quick meals when time is limited.

Make sure that you know the foods that contain the highest sodium content. It will help you to ensure that they are avoided entirely or they are limited in their use to prepare meals.

The foods to avoid are canned foods, rice mixes, condiments, salty snacks e.g. pretzels, pickled foods, pasta, frozen/ready-prepared meals, cheese, and deli meats which contains very high amounts of sodium.

For the packed food, check the labels for sodium content. What do you look out for? Check the label for the amount of sodium declared on the label. The sodium free foods contain less than 5mg of sodium per serving. Check for ingredients such as baking soda, bouillon cubes, broths, and condiments (e.g. mustard, ketchup, and barbecue sauce), baking powder, meat tenderizers, monosodium glutamate

High Blood Pressure

(MSG), dressings, sodium benzoate, soy sauce, and seasoned salts that are all high in salt.

These foods should be used in very small amounts if they must be used. Incidentally, the majority of these foods is low in nutrients and should be avoided.

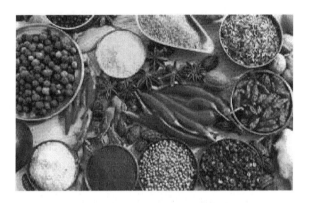

Fig: Alternative seasoning that can be used in place of salt

Learn to flavor or season food with spices other than salt. Not many people know that you can flavor food without salt. There are actually many options available through which to flavor food at home.

You can try options such as basil used on vegetables and lean meats e.g. chicken and fish, chili powder is good for stews, dried thyme which is also good for meats, and cumin. Other great seasoning options are dried and fresh rosemary, garlic, cinnamon, dried oregano, onions, parsley, fresh mint, ginger, and crushed red pepper.

High Blood Pressure

Shun directions provided in recipes to tailor make a dish that is low in sodium. Therefore, if the recipe calls for a pinch of salt, replace it with a herb of choice.

Reduce the intake of sodium by using smaller amount of salt in food and by even removing the salt shaker from the dinner table. Salt contributes to about ten percent of the total sodium intake. Salt is an acquired taste that can be gradually reduced to healthy levels. A 25 percent reduction in amount of salt used when preparing a meal will often go unnoticed.

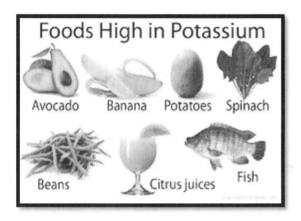

Fig: Examples of high potassium foods and vegetables

Eat a high amount of fruits and vegetables since they are high in potassium which helps to dull the impact of sodium in predisposing people to heart problems such high blood pressure. The potassium rich fruits and vegetables are bananas, dried apricots, kidney beans, melon, oranges, potatoes, and tomatoes.

High Blood Pressure

In conclusion, sodium is an essential nutrient required by the body for numerous functions but perhaps the most important is maintaining water balance in body cells. The daily sodium requirement of 500 milligrams should always be met but daily intake should never exceed 2300mg.

Too much sodium is an easier problem to fix than too little sodium in the body. Therefore, all attempts should be made to ensure that recommended daily dietary sodium level is met.

High Blood Pressure

Chapter 4

Meal planning

Meal planning for people with high blood pressure may seem an arduous task. But it is without doubt, a health saving measure that will prolong and preserve the quality of life.

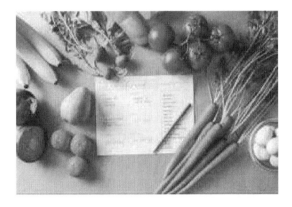

Fig: Meticulously plan your meals

A good strategy to adopt while preparing meals that are both nutritionally healthy and low in sodium level is that of the Plate Model. Creating the plate allows you to choose the food types that you want and beside that allows you to have the recommended portion sizes.

The plate model is best suited for the high blood pressure patients in their efforts to lower sodium intake and to maintain healthy body weight. it is characterized by a large amount of non-starchy vegetables that are rich in nutrients

High Blood Pressure

such as potassium that will counteract the effects of sodium from other food types. Half the plate will be filled with non-starchy vegetables such as greens, tomatoes, and carrots. Herbs and spices will added for extra flavor instead of salt. All the food should be prepared with healthy cooking methods such as roasting, grilling, steaming, or sautéing.

The following plan composed of seven steps will set you on the path to healthy low sodium diet.

i. With the use of the standard dinner plate, put a line down the middle of the plate. On one half of the plate, divide it into two to end up with a total of three parts on the plate.
ii. Fill the largest sector/section with non-starchy vegetables opting for fresh produce.
iii. In one of the two small sections, put grains and starchy foods that have low sodium levels.
iv. In the second small section, add your healthy proteins opting for lean meats such as chicken and fish.
v. Add a serving of fruit to the meal plan.
vi. Choose healthy fats in small amounts both for cooking and in your salads.
vii. To complete the meal, add a low-calorie drink like water, unsweetened tea or coffee.

When planning meals, always keep in mind that practically any recipe can easily be made into a low sodium recipe. The first planning step is to know and start eliminating processed foods that contain extremely high sodium levels.

High Blood Pressure

These foods contain high levels of sodium which is used as a preservative.

- Buy fresh fruits and vegetables instead of going for the canned veggies.
- Buy fresh poultry, fish and meat instead of processed or smoked varieties
- Cook brown rice instead of instant or flavored or pre-processed types.
- Cook whole baked potatoes instead of instant or flavored potatoes.
- Rinse canned foods such as tuna to strip off the high sodium fluid in which they are preserved.

Another planning step is to find alternative to common salt used to add flavor to food. Find a good tasting salt substitute that does not contain sodium or potassium chloride that carries a metallic taste. Use fresh seasonings e.g. parsley, tomatoes, mint, rosemary since seasonings lose their flavor or get a get a flavor change when they start getting old. You will be looking to get the maximum natural flavor from the chosen seasoning.

High Blood Pressure

Chapter 5

Breakfast

Low sodium breakfast should be the way to start the day for patients with high blood pressure. The diets are also the best way to commence the day for middle aged adults as well as seniors who happen to be at high risk of high blood pressure and other heart diseases.

The general idea is to limit the inclusion of processed meats, butter and salted egg dishes that contain a high amount of sodium. Subtle changes to the preparation of breakfast will make it healthy and containing low amounts of sodium.

Choose low-sodium varieties of meat or make your own breakfast meat. The processed breakfast meats such as sausage and bacon contain extremely high quantities of sodium.

Avoid the bread and cereal products sold off the shelf since they contain sodium based preservatives. Instead use homemade oatmeal as well as making your own homemade pastries and baked products without adding salt as a breakfast item.

Choose unsalted butter or use polyunsaturated or monounsaturated oils to prepare a low sodium breakfast. For dairy products, use low fat milk and low fat yogurt and low sodium cheese. Eggs should be prepared without the

High Blood Pressure

addition of salt preferring to use herbs and spices such as onion and garlic.

Finally, add fresh fruit and fresh vegetables that are low in sodium to your breakfast. Include fruit slices and vegetables such as spinach to smoothies, omelets, and pancakes to enrich your breakfast.

Examples of the good breakfast recipes are:

Grandpa Hubbard's Oatmeal

Ingredients

- 3/4 cups water
- 1/4 cup brown sugar
- 2 cups rolled oats
- 4 teaspoons butter
- 1 pinch salt
- 4 tablespoons milk
- 1/4 cup brown sugar
- 1 cup non-dairy creamer

Directions

1. In a medium saucepan, heat water to boiling. Reduce heat to low; stir in oats and salt. Cook until oats have thickened, about 5 minutes.

2. Place 1 teaspoon of butter and 1 tablespoon of brown sugar in the bottom of each four serving bowls. Spoon oatmeal into each bowl and stir until butter and

High Blood Pressure

sugar are melted. Pour 1/4 cup of creamer and 1 tablespoon of milk over each bowl. Top each serving with another tablespoon of brown sugar. Serve hot.

Total time taken to prepare is 30 minutes

Popovers

Ingredients

- 2 tablespoons unsalted butter, chilled
- 1 cup all-purpose flour
- 3 eggs
- 1/4 teaspoon salt
- 1 tablespoon unsalted butter, melted
- 1 cup milk

Directions

1. Preheat oven to 220 degrees C.

2. Spray a popover pan with nonstick cooking spray. Place pan on center rack of oven and preheat for 2 minutes.

3. Blend flour, salt, eggs, milk, and melted butter until it looks like heavy cream, about 1 to 2 minutes.

4. Cut chilled butter into 6 even pieces. Place 1 piece of butter in each cup and place pan back in oven until butter is bubbly (about 1 minute).

5. Fill each cup half full with batter and bake 20 minutes. Reduce heat to 325 degrees F (165 degrees C) and bake for another 15 to 20 minutes.

Total time taken to prepare is 2 hours.

Chapter 6

Lunch and Dinner

The same principle of reducing the levels of sodium intake that applies for breakfast also applies for lunch and dinner. The food choices made should bypass the processed foods that have high quantities of sodium.

Here are a few examples of low sodium recipes that will greatly benefit patients with high blood pressure.

Hamburger Buddy

Served with green salad, the hamburger buddy can make a good meal for lunch or supper.

Ingredients (6 servings)

- 3 cloves garlic, crushed and peeled
- 1 tablespoon chopped fresh parsley, or chives for garnish
- 2 medium carrots, cut into 2-inch pieces
- 1 pound 90%-lean ground beef
- 10 ounces white mushrooms, large ones cut in half

High Blood Pressure

- 1 large onion, cut into 2-inch pieces
- 8 ounces whole-wheat elbow noodles, (2 cups)
- 2 teaspoons dried thyme
- 3/4 teaspoon salt
- 2 tablespoons all-purpose flour
- 1/4 teaspoon freshly ground pepper
- 1 14-ounce can reduced-sodium beef broth, divided
- 2 cups water
- 2 tablespoons Worcestershire sauce
- 1/2 cup reduced-fat sour cream

Preparation

Total Preparation Time = 1 hour 20 minutes

    i   Using a food processor fitted with a steel blade attachment, finely mince garlic before adding carrots and mushrooms until they are finely chopped. The onions and pulse are then roughly chopped.

    ii   Cook beef in a large straight-sided skillet or Dutch oven over medium-high heat, breaking it up with a wooden spoon. Stir in the chopped vegetables, thyme, salt and pepper and cook until the vegetables start to soften and the mushrooms release their juices.

    iii   While stirring, add water, 1 1/2 cups broth, noodles and Worcestershire sauce; bring to a boil. Cover the skillet; reduce heat to medium and cook, stirring occasionally until the pasta is tender. It will take 8 to 10 minutes.

iv Whisk flour with the remaining 1/4 cup broth in a small bowl and add it into the hamburger mixture while stirring. Stir in the sour cream and simmer until the sauce has thickened. Serve sprinkled with parsley.

Chicken & Spinach Soup with Fresh Pesto

It makes use of a boneless and skinless chicken breast as well as baby spinach and canned beans.

Ingredients for 5 servings

- 1 large boneless, skinless chicken breast cut into quarters
- 5 cups reduced-sodium chicken broth
- 2 teaspoons plus 1 tablespoon extra-virgin olive oil
- 1/2 cup carrot or diced red bell pepper
- 1 large clove garlic, minced
- 1 15-ounce can cannellini beans or great northern beans, rinsed
- 1 1/2 teaspoons dried marjoram
- 6 ounces baby spinach, coarsely chopped
- Freshly ground pepper to taste
- 1/4 cup grated Parmesan cheese
- 1/3 cup lightly packed fresh basil leaves

High Blood Pressure

Preparation

Total Preparation Time = 1 hour

i. Heat 2 teaspoons oil in a large saucepan or Dutch oven over medium-high heat. Add carrot/bell pepper and chicken; cook while stirring frequently and turning the chicken, until it begins to brown.

ii. Add garlic while stirring and cook for 1 minute. Thereafter, stir in broth and marjoram and bring it to boil over high heat. Reduce the heat and simmer for about 5 minutes, stirring occasionally until the chicken is well cooked.

iii. Using a slotted spoon, remove the chicken pieces and allow them to cool on a clean cutting board. Add the spinach and beans to the pot and bring to a gentle boil. Cook for 5 minutes to blend in the flavors.

iv. Combine the remaining 1 tablespoon oil, Parmesan and basil in a food processor and process while adding a little water and scraping down the sides as necessary until a coarse paste forms,.

v. Cut the chicken into bite-size pieces. Stir the chicken and pesto into the pot. Season with pepper and cook until hot.

High Blood Pressure

Chapter 7

Dessert

The following recipes will create good desserts that are best suited for hypertensive patients.

Peanut Butter & Pretzel Truffles

The peanut butter-pretzel truffles are just the best choice for sating the craving for sweet and salty flavors.

Ingredients for 20 servings

- 1/2 cup crunchy natural peanut butter
- 1/2 cup milk chocolate chips
- 1/4 cup finely chopped salted pretzels

Preparation

Total Preparation time = 2 hours and 15 minutes

i. Mix the peanut butter and pretzels in a small bowl. Then, chill for 15 minutes in the freezer to make it firm.

ii. Roll the peanut butter mixture into 20 balls (about 1 teaspoon each). Place on a baking sheet lined with wax paper and freeze until very firm for about 1 hour.

iii. Take out the frozen balls and roll them in melted chocolate. Refrigerate until the chocolate is set, about 30 minutes.

High Blood Pressure

Kale Chips

Ingredients for 4 servings

- 1 large bunch kale, tough stems removed and leaves torn into pieces.
- 1 tablespoon extra-virgin olive oil
- 1/4 teaspoon salt

Preparation

Total Preparation time = 50 minutes

i.   Position racks in upper third and center of oven, and preheat the oven to 400°F.

ii.   In a large bowl, sprinkle the kale with oil and sprinkle with salt. Using your hands, massage the oil and salt onto the kale leaves to evenly coat. Fill large rimmed baking sheets with a layer of kale, making sure the leaves don't overlap.

iii.   Bake until most leaves are crisp, 8 to 12 minutes in total.

High Blood Pressure

Chapter 8

40 Super Foods That Will Naturally Lower Your Blood Pressure

High blood pressure can be tackled via a number of methods that include relaxing, exercising regularly, sleeping more, taking medications daily, and changing eating habits.

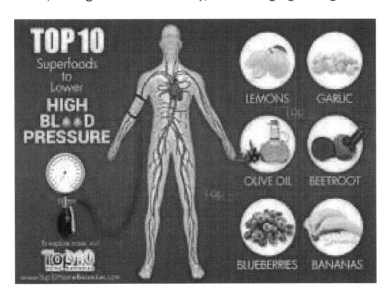

Fig: Some of the superfoods to help manage high blood pressure

Altering eating habits is perhaps the most difficult of them all. However, it must be done to improve your cardiovascular health and to increase life span. There are numerous foods that can help to lower blood pressure naturally.

High Blood Pressure

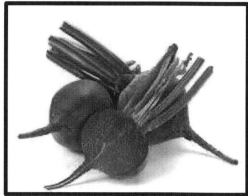

1. Beetroot contains nitrates and nitrites which can be converted into nitric oxide in the body. Nitric oxide signals the cells in the walls of your arteries to relax and soften. The effect is that it improves vasodilation and lowers blood pressure.

2. Yogurt is a good source of nutrients such as potassium, magnesium and calcium that enable you to keep your blood pressure in check.

3. Garlic contains allicin, a sulphur compound that significantly lowers elevated blood pressure. A study has indicated that garlic is as effective as prescribed medications after 24 weeks.

4. Fish oil contains omega-3 fatty acids that are extremely beneficial to the health of the human cardiovascular system. The omega 3 fats have been found to effective only seen in people with existing hypertension.

High Blood Pressure

5. Cashews and Almonds are rich magnesium will protect against blood pressure and associated complications.

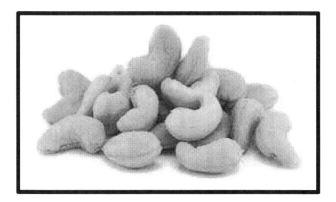

Fig: Cashew nuts

Numerous studies have shown that replacing the lack of magnesium greatly reduces high blood pressure.

6. Kale is yet another superfood and is loaded with vitamins, minerals, antioxidants, and other compounds known to help prevent disease. Kale is particularly rich in both magnesium and potassium, a combination that strongly linked to lower blood pressure levels in high blood pressure.

7. Stevia, a natural sweetener contains the active compound stevioside that was found to decrease systolic blood pressure by 8.1 percent and diastolic blood pressure by 13.8 percent after three months in study participants who had high blood pressure.

High Blood Pressure

8. Turmeric contains an active ingredient called curcumin that has powerful anti-inflammatory effects in the body.

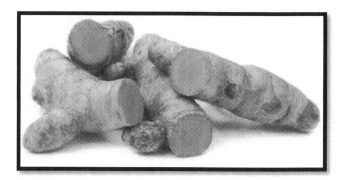

Fig: Turmeric contains curcumin that protects against high blood pressure

Curcumin has been found to successfully improve blood flow levels akin to people who exercise three times per week. The benefits of curcumin on blood flow and blood pressure are related to nitric oxide similar to what we have noted with beetroot.

9. Green tea is laden with powerful compounds and antioxidants. One such compound is catechin that improves blood flow and blood pressure. Consuming two cups of green tea each day will lead to a 40 percent increase in arterial diameter effectively reducing blood pressure.

High Blood Pressure

10. Tomatoes have been shown through research to help with blood pressure problems. It is best to eat tomatoes close to raw, without much processing or cooking to get the best out of them.

11. Green coffee retains chlorogenic acid which has a short term benefit in aiding blood flow. A study shows that green coffee reduces heart rate and blood pressure by about 8 percent and this is retained only for 12 weeks.

12. Spinach is another vegetable that is packed with nutrients and antioxidants that help the body to repair damage caused by stress.

13. Extra-virgin olive oil is perhaps the healthiest oil in the world. It is rich in heart-friendly monounsaturated fats and phenolic antioxidants.

High Blood Pressure

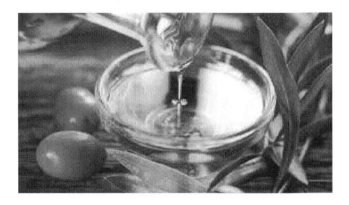

Fig: Olive oil protects against heart diseases

The oil reduces heart attacks, strokes, and death by a staggering 30 percent. Olive oil could therefore cut the need for blood pressure medications.

14. Hibiscus tea also known as roselle tea or sour tea contains anthocyanins and is proven to reduce high blood pressure. A study has revealed that consuming a large cup of hibiscus tea before breakfast each day for 4 weeks is associated with reductions of 11 percent in systolic pressure and 12.5 percent reduction in diastolic blood pressure.

15. Raisins are a fantastic snack in between meals. Raisins have a high amount of potassium that is good for the heart. To reap the maximum health benefits from potassium, eat the raw and natural raisins without added sugars.

High Blood Pressure

16. Pomegranates are a good source of artery relaxing nitrates can lower blood pressure and improve other heart health markers.

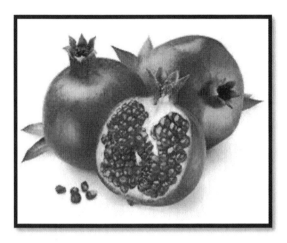

Fig: Pomegranates help to relax the arteries

Relaxed arteries are soft and elastic therefore they do not cause resistance to blood flow. Taking pomegranate juice daily for 2 weeks can markedly lower both systolic and diastolic blood pressure.

17. Potatoes and sweet potatoes are rich in potassium which works in tandem with sodium to regulate the electrical activity of the heart. Studies carried out indicate that increased potassium intake significantly reduces high blood pressure except for those with chronic kidney disease.

High Blood Pressure

18. Mushrooms contain an active ingredient called ergothioneine, a powerful antioxidant that helps to protect arterial cells from oxidative damage.

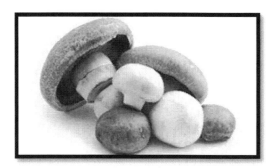

Fig: Mushrooms contain ergothioneine that prevents high blood pressure

Ergothioneine appears to protect and preserve nitric oxide which is fundamental to healthy blood flow and pressure.

19. Dark chocolate contain flavanols that help to inhibit angiotensin converting enzyme (ACE) thereby lowering blood pressure. The really dark chocolates (with up to 85 percent cocoa) contain 25 to 40 grams of flavanols.

20. Fermented foods contain a not so common vitamin called menaquinone or vitamin K2 that improves vascular health. The foods with the highest amount of vitamin K2 are animal products such as dairy products, meat and egg yolks as well as fermented foods such as sauerkraut, natto and miso. Vitamin

High Blood Pressure

K2 inhibits the progression of arterial stiffness which in turn preserves cardiovascular health.

21. The fermented foods also provide gut bacteria with probiotics. Healthy gut bacteria have been linked to lower blood pressure through kidney regulation.

22. Herring, salmon and other fatty fish species are good for the heart since they are good sources of coenzyme Q10 (CoQ10) also referred to as ubiquinone. Ubiquinone is an antioxidant and is good for cells that are involved with blood flow hence leading to healthy blood pressure levels. These types of fish are also good sources of omega 3 fats and potassium which are good for the heart.

23. Spirulina is blue - green type of algae that grows in both fresh and salt water has been shown to lower blood pressure.

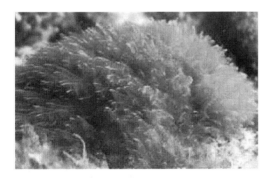

Fig: Spirulina is a superfood and is known to protect against heart disease

High Blood Pressure

Spirulina contains high levels of the signaling molecule nitric oxide which helps to improve cardiovascular health and prevent high blood pressure. Spirulina can thus be used by people with high blood pressure to lower blood pressure.

24. Apples contain high levels of oligomeric proanthocyanidins (OPCs) which are able to aid healthy blood circulation, to boost the health of veins, and reduce blood pressure levels. A good example of the OPCs is quercetin that lowers blood pressure.

25. Onions are also good sources of oligomeric proanthocyanidins which can help hypertensive patients to lower blood pressure. The onions can be combined with other foods such as garlic and olive oil that are also heart healthy and support healthy blood circulation.

26. Prunes are good natural food for maintaining healthy blood pressure levels. Prunes are known to reduce the levels of bad cholesterol effectively lowering blood pressure.

27. Natto is a fermented soy product that appears like cheese. The soy is first boiled and then fermented with *Bacillus subtilis natto* and can be served with foods such as salads and cabbage. Nattokinase the active ingredient in natto is a naturally remedy for high blood pressure. However, people who have

High Blood Pressure

been put on Coumadin, a blood thinning medication should not consume natto.

28. Flaxseed can be crushed and consumed together with breakfast cereals to maintain healthy blood pressure levels.

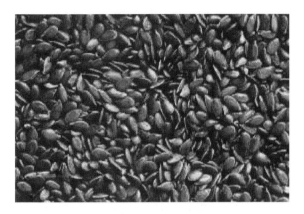

Fig: Flaxseed is quite helpful in managing blood pressure

Flaxseed contains two types of essential fatty acids namely omega-6 fats and alpha linolenic acid, the precursor for omega-3 fats.

29. Avocados contain the healthy monounsaturated fats such as the omega-3 fats that stimulate the production of nitric oxide. Nitric oxide keeps arteries properly dilated, and counteracts the vasoconstricting effect of stress that can cause high blood pressure.

30. Potatoes contain a compound known as kukoamine that may potentially lower blood pressure.

High Blood Pressure

31. Wakame, a type of seaweed popular in Japan is good for heart health.

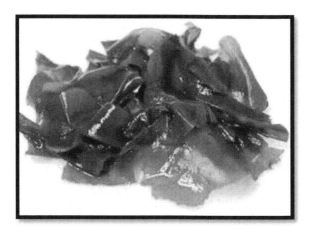

Fig: Wakame is common in Japan and is helpful for people with hypertension

It has been indicated that taking about 3 grams of dried wakame over a period of four weeks helped to reduce systolic blood pressure by up to 14 points and diastolic blood pressure by up to 5 points.

32. *Ecklonia cava,* an edible Asian red-brown alga, has been discovered to contain natural plant compounds that help dilate blood vessels and act as a natural remedy for high blood pressure.

High Blood Pressure

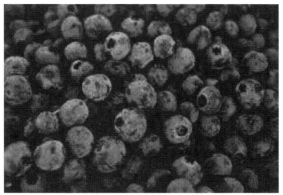

33. Blueberres have high levels of antioxidants that really aid heart health and healthy blood pressure. Blueberries can be a good breakfast option for people with high blood pressure.

34. Green beans are a good source of vitamin C, fiber and potassium all of which are good for your heart and will lower your blood pressure.

35. Carrots are a good source of antioxidants and potassium which are two major supporters of normal blood pressure levels.

High Blood Pressure

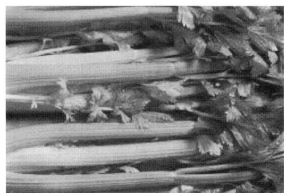

36. Celery contains apigenin that has properties that promote relaxing of blood vessels and lowering of blood pressure. Celery in all its forms will therefore act as a natural remedy for high blood pressure.

37. Peas are a good source of vitamins and folic acid, providing overall cardiovascular support, making them a perfect food to prevent high blood pressure.

38. Papaya is an incredible source of vitamin C, amino acids and potassium that all contribute to a healthy heart and lower blood pressure levels.

39. Kiwi fruits can help to keep blood pressure from becoming a problem.

High Blood Pressure

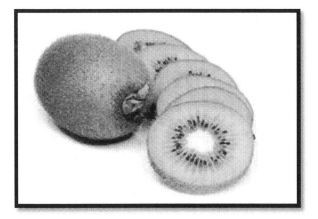

Fig: Kiwi fruit has numerous benefits including preventing hypertension

Research has shown that eating three kiwis a day will protect individuals from high blood pressure.

40. Watermelon is a wondrous fruit and contains L-citrulline which helps relax the arteries leading to lower blood pressure levels.

41. Sweet potatoes contain glutathione, an antioxidant that can protect against high blood pressure, heart attack, and stroke.

High Blood Pressure

Chapter 9

Bonus Juicing Recipes

Making use of the superfoods alongside other nutritious vegetables and fruits, hypertensive patients can benefit from natural juice recipes that lower blood pressure and prevent adverse heart disease.

The following are good examples of juicing recipes that lower blood pressure.

Beet Celery Apple Juice

Ingredients

- 1 beet
- 4 Stalks celery
- Half an inch ginger
- 1 Small apple

Directions

i. Wash all vegetables.
ii. Keep skin on veggies and apple as much as possible.
iii. Juice and enjoy.

Antioxidant Supreme

Ingredients

High Blood Pressure

- 1 cup fresh blueberries
- 1 cup (about 5) fresh strawberries
- 2 cups peeled and coarsely chopped mango
- 1/4 cup of water

Preparation

i. Combine the blueberries, strawberries, mango, and water in a blender.
ii. Blend while occasionally scraping down sides until smooth.
iii. Strain juice and, if desired, thin with additional water.
iv. Refrigerate up to 2 days (shake before serving).

Turmeric Sunrise

Ingredients

- 2 medium apples
- 3 medium carrots
- 3 large stalks of celery
- 1 thumb of ginger
- 2 lemons (peeled)
- 2 medium pears
- 6 thumbs of turmeric Root

Preparation

Process all ingredients in a juicer, shake or stir and serve.

Chapter 10

Relaxing Techniques

Relaxation techniques are part of the natural ways through which people can manage high blood pressure. People can explore these techniques to help them relax and deal with stress.

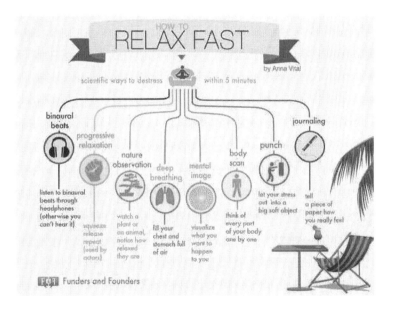

Fig: Relaxation techniques that will help keep off stress and maintain health blood pressure

Stress is a major cause of vasoconstriction and high blood pressure. Relaxation techniques usually help people to cope with everyday stress and with stress caused by other health problems such as pain.

High Blood Pressure

It should be remembered that the relaxation techniques are not only about enjoying a hobby or peace of mind. By relaxing, people benefit from a process that decreases the effects of stress on the mind and the body.

Relaxation techniques are either free or low cost and can be done just about anywhere. Learning the basic relaxation techniques is quite straightforward. The techniques are not associated with any major risks.

We have a look at the relaxation techniques that can be of great benefit for people with high blood pressure.

- Autogenic relaxation makes use of both visual imagery and body awareness to reduce stress. Autogenic in this case means that is it something that comes from inside of you.

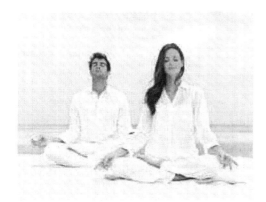

Fig: Autogenic breathing exercises

An illustration of how the technique works is imagining a peaceful and beautiful setting and then

High Blood Pressure

focusing on controlled, relaxing breathing. You can repeat words or suggestions you have crafted in your mind to relax and reduce muscle tension. The effects are that the heart rate slows and you feel different physical sensations, such as relaxing each arm or leg one by one.

- Visualization involves the formation of mental images that will usher you into a peaceful, calming place or situation.

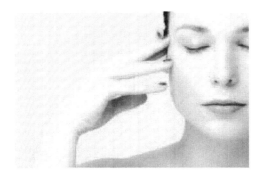

Fig: Visualization techniques bring about peace of mind

It is recommended that during visualization, you should try to use as many senses as you can, including the senses of smell, sound, sight, and touch. For example, when you imagine relaxing by the ocean, think about the smell of salty ocean water, the sound of breaking waves and the warmth of the sun on your skin.

- Meditation is the practice of focusing on an object or a single point of awareness.

High Blood Pressure

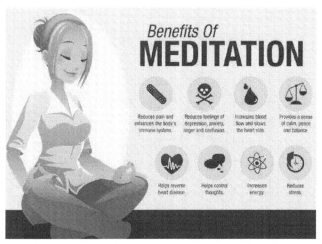

Fig: Benefits of meditation include improving blood flow

Regular practice of meditation can give you calm and oneness, stillness of mind, inner peace, happiness and emotional stability, heightened clarity, improved concentration and focus, increased vitality and rejuvenation, improved memory and learning ability.

Meditation decreases the negative effects of stress, anxiety and depression. In so doing, meditation leads to a reduction in the probability of experiencing any heart related illnesses.

- Yoga is a common discipline that allows people to practice meditation as well as exercise. The type of

High Blood Pressure

yoga you choose to practice is entirely an individual preference.

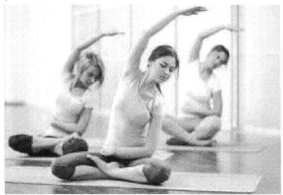

Fig: Yoga is both a type of relaxation and exercise that benefits the cardiovascular system

The differences lie in fact that some hold the postures longer whereas others move through the postures quicker. Some styles focus on body alignment, others differ in the rhythm and selection of postures, meditation and spiritual realization.

You should therefore choose the Yoga style dependent on individual psychological and physical needs. In our case, yoga styles that focus on helping manage high blood pressure.

Other types of relaxation techniques are:

- Biofeedback
- Hypnosis
- Massage
- Deep breathing

High Blood Pressure

- Tai chi
- Music and art therapy

Overall the benefits of relaxation to high blood pressure patients include:

a) Lowering blood pressure
b) Slowing your heart rate
c) Reducing activity of stress hormones
d) Increasing blood flow to major muscles
e) Slowing your breathing rate

View more books from

ARNOLD YATES

Bodybuilding: How to Easily Build Muscles and Keep Mass Permanently: 10X your Results and Build the Physique That You Want.

Atkins Diet: Lose Weight and Feel Great, Contains Tips and Recipes

Calisthenics for Beginners: A Beginners guide to body weight training

High Blood Pressure

Conclusion

Blood pressure is perhaps the best indicator of overall cardiovascular health. People with high blood pressure are often at a significantly greater risk for chronic kidney disease, heart failure, stroke, and damage to the arteries which can cause heart attack.

Managing and preventing high blood pressure isn't an option. The two tasks call for understanding the causes and making smart decisions about factors under your control.

The most effective and sustainable measure for preventing and managing hypertension is through lifestyle changes. It is however not an easy task compared to popping a pill.

Perhaps, the most important thing is that you must find the personal motivation and the required determination to see through the necessary lifestyle changes. Prevention is better than cure.

High Blood Pressure

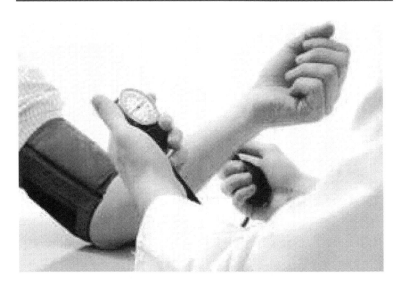

Fig: Regular blood pressure checks will help prevent high blood pressure

Lastly, regular visits to your doctor will ensure that early diagnosis and management of high blood pressure. The visits to the doctor should be made even if you feel generally healthy. The doctor will help to identify risk factors in the situation that you do not have the disease and recommend lifestyle changes to prevent onset. Remember that high blood pressure is also referred to as the silent killer since it may go unnoticed for very long.

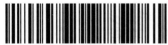

Made in the USA
Middletown, DE
18 January 2017